LIFE as a NURSE

20 plus years –

seen, heard, done,

and said so many things……

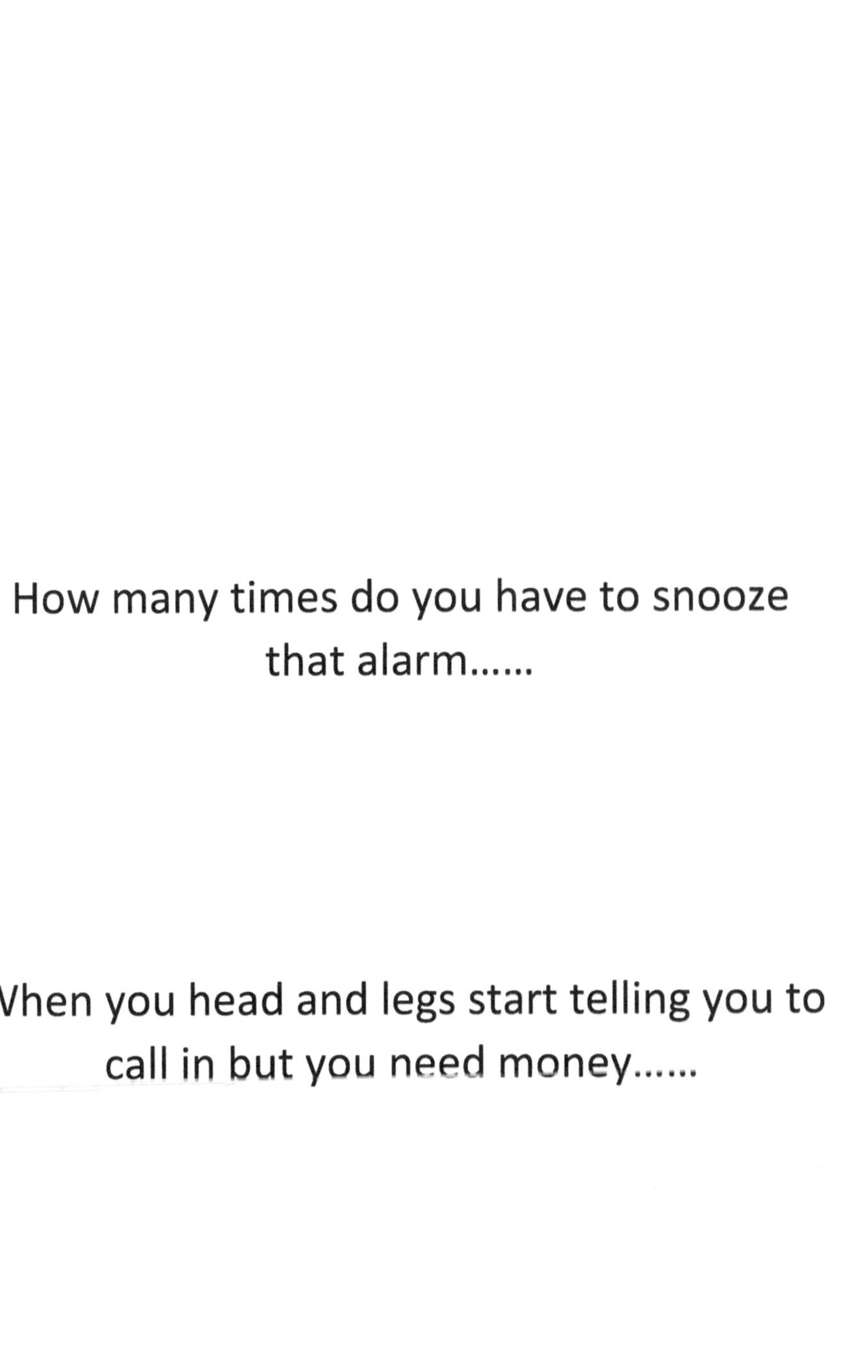
How many times do you have to snooze
that alarm......

When you head and legs start telling you to
call in but you need money......

When you put your scrubs on in the morning and your body already hurts…..

That long drive through traffic …………

Then you arrive and it all begins here........
Memories to last you a life time!!!

Getting asked questions and questions and questions when you haven't even clocked in or have name badge on, or even feel like talking....

Looking at the schedule to see what unit you assigned.... Long-term, ICU, mental and substance abuse, therapy, ER, surgical, nursery, skilled, etc... so you can mentally prepare yourself.....

Who are your working with ...... favorite coworker, friend, enemy, busy bees, lazy staff, brown nose, late staff, no staff.......

Getting report who did this, who did that, who didn't take this med, who took to many meds ,who fell, who walked out , left AMA, admissions, discharges, what, where , how   and why……

Then you see snacks, cookie, tacos, candy at nurse station is it time for a sugar rush   or not yet…..

Call lights ringing, cannot find aids, or any staff, lost your notes, food trays need to be passed out, someone yelling for help, someone yelling in pain ,computer has just locked you out, password expired, naked patient in hall……. Let the day begin welcome to being a NURSE   got to LOVE it, wouldn't change it for the world.

Your blood pressure cuff   need batteries, the vital sign machine is broken, nail polish on the nail for the pulse off, your watch does not have second hand. Small work blockers or not.....

Going down the hall way -Med cart wheels turn the wrong way,   med cart heavy as hell!, drawers stuck, missing   medicine, sticky liquids left uncovered, spills in cart, expired medicine, undated medicine, pill crusher broken, empty medicine OTC bottles. No ice or water pitchers,   the list goes on..

Keys, keys, where are the keys, wrong pocket ……

Pen, Marker, paper, highlighter, scissors………ready!!

Room 101A   knock, knock   anybody here??

Hello there?, how are you today?, may I check your vital signs?, are you in a good mood? Have you eaten? Have you had a bowel movement? Pain? Please don't stare at me that way, are you going to kick me out or will you take your pills, (thoughts in my head)

Charting- was that this patient or the other, who got what, when, where, and why. Who needs this and that, Notes, Notes where my notes…… my pen running out of ink… of course it would

Looking up at clock…. How many hours, minutes, seconds…. Till I go to lunch, home or even pee!!!

And somebody is in the restroom!!

Walking down the hall, checking patients as you walk by, tripping on you crocs! Checking for keys are in pocket, heading for snack machine... I need a break until that snack machine is out of order, or keeps your money with nothing in return, or has nothing good you like to snack on.

Walking back to nurses station and everybody looking for you like you have been gone forever , all you did was go get a snack (maybe), saying so and so needs this and that,   this don't work that don't work .

Composure- smile - how can I help you ?

Sitting at nurses station Finally when   ring, ring ,ring ,ring, ring, ring – (hoping it will stop) admission- please get report, family member how is so and so, pharmacy how much supply is left, or patient calling themselves please come to my room.....

The big RING,RING, RING   fire alarm drill, get up , secure residents, close doors, let everyone know it's a drill before they panic, do I lock myself in a room or start looking for fire extinguisher   - you know it's the monthly drill. It will be ok   where do I sign……

Now can I go eat lunch…….   Or what's next..

Lunch is here

Forgot my locker key in car to far to go get.

Eating my soggy, cold lunch, for yesterday that I had in my bag or door dasher got the wrong order again, break room gossip don't want to be involved, can't help but listen. Or TV news   on- please bring world peace!!

Restroom break- no toilet-paper, no
napkins , no soap,   shake it off or air dry
decisions, decisions, can even get a break
on break

Back to floor - knowing day half way
through pleased let this be a smooth ride
downhill, lets finish what needs to be done

Treatment- wounds, cuts, abrasion, pus, blood, gangrene, smelly, drainage either you love it or hate it, it has to be done let's get to it

Treatment cart not stocked, just put a band aid!! That should do the trick for now or for a couple of seconds……. Of to supply room I go

Medicine   done

Treatment done

Assessment done

Patient round done

Orders done

Charting... emmm   almost done

Time is getting closer , I can almost feel the sun on my face driving home, then I realized I need to stop at grocery – get dinner for tonight , and put gas   since I am on empty and to sleepy to stop this morning…..

And of course a patient falls , seems about right almost end of shift , well excuse me this nurse has a job to do……. Besides that's what I am here for   now let me start on assessment and paper work so I can get out on time….

Done relaxing   feet starting to hurt, why
did I wear these shoes, theses tight scubs,

Maybe now I can go peee!

What a relief !!!   my bladder thanks me, I
feel skinner , lighter .

Clock says   my shift is over!!! Lets wrap it
up

Waiting on relief   the longest wait ever,
seems like an eternity   but that smile on my
face knowing they walked in the building
and are about to clock in

The drive home or HEB or valero - thinking of everything I did and still need to be done.....
follow ups ... did I forget this that, did I say this that...... I am sure I did

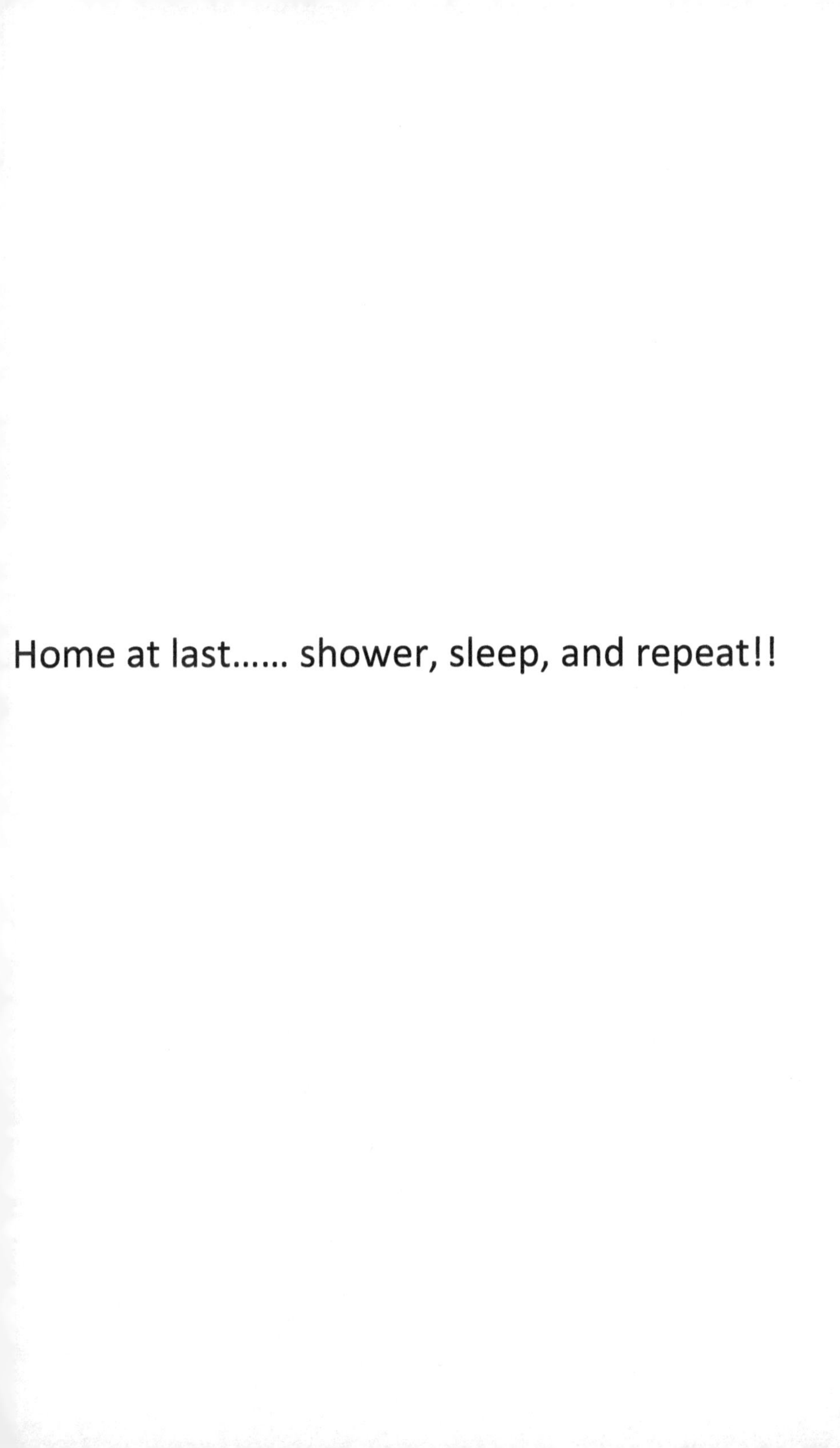
Home at last…… shower, sleep, and repeat!!

www.ingramcontent.com/pod-product-compliance
Lightning Source LLC
Chambersburg PA
CBHW051240250726
48656CB00003B/1048